ANDERSON JEFFREY MD

MIGRAINES:

An Overview Of Primary Headaches

Contents

1.

2.

3.

4.

5.

6.

7.

8.

9.

10.

11.

12.

13.

14.

15.

1

INTRODUCTION

How are migraines assessed and analyzed?

Assuming you have cerebral pains frequently or on the other hand on the off chance that they are extremely serious, contact your medical services supplier. You can generally begin with your family doctor, where the conclusion cycle will start. It's vital to analyze migraines accurately so unambiguous treatment can be begun to assist you with feeling improved.

Your medical care supplier will finish an actual assessment, examine your clinical history and converse with you about your migraine side effects. This discussion is important for a cerebral pain assessment.

During the cerebral pain assessment, your supplier will get some information about your migraine history, including:

A depiction of your migraines.

What the migraines feel like.

How frequently the migraines occur.

How long the migraines last each time.

How much torment the migraines cause you.

What food sources, beverages or occasions trigger your cerebral pains.

How much caffeine you drink every day.

What your feeling of anxiety are.

What your rest propensities are like.

Assuming you have any work issues.

Your cerebral pain can be all the more precisely analyzed by knowing:

At the point when the migraine began.

How long you have had the cerebral pain.

Whether there is a solitary kind of cerebral pain or numerous sorts of migraines.

How frequently the migraine happens.

What causes the migraine, whenever known (for instance, do specific circumstances, food sources, or prescriptions normally trigger the cerebral pain?).

Assuming active work irritates the migraine torment.

What occasions are related with the cerebral pain.

Who else in your family has migraines.

What side effects, if any, happen between cerebral pains.

Your primary care physician will likewise pose extra inquiries about execution at work, family foundation, and assuming there is any set of experiences of substance addiction.

Clinical portrayal of migraines

Portray how you feel when you have the migraine and what happens when you get the cerebral pain, for example,

Where the aggravation is found.

What it seems like.

How extreme the migraine torment is, utilizing a scale from 1 (gentle) to 10 (serious).

On the off chance that the cerebral pain shows up out of nowhere abruptly or with going with side effects.

What season of day the migraine normally happens.

Assuming that there is a quality (changes in vision, vulnerable sides, or splendid lights) before the cerebral pain.

What different side effects or cautioning signs happen with the migraine (shortcoming, queasiness, aversion to light or clamor, diminished hunger, changes in mentality or conduct).

HOW LONG THE MIGRAINE ENDURES

History of Migraine Medicines

You ought to furnish your doctor with a background marked by earlier migraine medicines.

Let your primary care physician know what drugs you have taken before and what medication are you right now taking. Make sure to them, get the medicine bottles or ask your drug specialist for a printout.

If any examinations or tests were recently performed, carry them with you. This might save time and redundancy of tests.

Physical and neurological assessments for migraines

In the wake of finishing the clinical history part of the assessment, your doctor will carry out physical and neurological assessments. The doctor will search for signs and side effects of a sickness that might be causing the cerebral pain.

These signs and side effects can include:

Fever

Disease

Hypertension

Muscle shortcoming, deadness, or shivering

Unnecessary weariness, needing to rest constantly

Loss of awareness

Balance issues, falling

Vision issues (hazy vision, twofold vision, vulnerable sides)

Mental disarray or changes in character, unseemly way of behaving, discourse hardships

Seizures

Dazedness

Sickness, retching

Neurological tests center around precluding sicknesses that could likewise cause migraines, like epilepsy, different sclerosis, and other cerebrovascular infections. An issue of the focal sensory system may be associated in the improvement with serious migraines.

These include:

Cancer

Sore

Discharge (draining inside the cerebrum)

Bacterial or viral meningitis (a contamination or irritation of the layer that covers the mind and spinal line)

Pseudotumor cerebri (expanded intracranial tension)

Hydrocephalus (unusual development of liquid in the cerebrum)

Contamination of the cerebrum

Encephalitis (aggravation of the cerebrum)

Blood clumps

Head injury

Sinus blockage or sickness

Mutation (like Arnold-Chiari)

Wounds

Contamination, like Lyme sickness

Meningitis

Aneurysm

In the wake of assessing the consequences of your cerebral pain history, actual assessment and neurological assessment, your doctor ought to have the option to figure out what kind of migraine you have, whether a difficult issue is available and whether extra tests are required.

On the off chance that conceivable, attempt to record how you feel when you are encountering a migraine. Keeping a diary of your cerebral pains and how they affect you can be useful when you are conversing with your medical services supplier.

The data you give your medical services supplier about your cerebral pains is the main piece of the analysis cycle.

By giving your supplier however much data as could reasonably be expected about your migraines, you're bound to get a precise determination and a treatment plan that will assist you with feeling improved.

Despite the fact that sweeps and other envisioning tests can be significant while precluding different illnesses, they don't help in diagnosing headaches, bunch or pressure type cerebral pains.

Nonetheless, assuming your medical care supplier feels that your cerebral pains are being brought about by one more ailment, there are a few imaging tests that might be finished.

A CT output or X-ray can be utilized in the event that your supplier thinks your cerebral pains are associated with an issue with your focal sensory system.

Both of these tests produce cross-sectional pictures of the cerebrum that can show any unusual regions or issues. X-beams of your skull are for the most part not done. An EEG (electroencephalogram) may not be required except if you've at any point dropped during a migraine.

There's perhaps no medical terminology/condition— save for the "malarias," and the "typhoids"—
as abused as "migraine" by the uninitiated.

Migraine has come to mean different things to different people: for some, it is any headache that is "severe" and perhaps incapacitating. To others, it is any headache that recurs habitually.

With this lose definition of the term migraine, fact is that many headache syndromes labeled as "migraines" are not actually migraines.

In this book, we will be looking at the different types of primary headaches, including those often mistaken by the uninitiated as "migraines," and the typical migraine headaches.

2

HEADACHES: Primary Vs. Secondary

Headaches **are broadly classified into Primary and Secondary forms:**

✓ Primary headaches are headache syndromes which are disease entities of their own; they are usually nor caused by some other illness.

✓ Secondary headaches are those that arise as part of the symptoms of another illness; they are therefore caused by a readily identifiable local, or systemic illness.

Example of causes of secondary headaches include;

- Malaria

- Typhoid

- Hypertension

- Sinusitis

- Brain tumor

- Meningitis

- Brain bleed.

-   Etc.

3

PRIMARY HEADACHES, and MIGRAINES

Primary headaches, as hinted above, are headache syndromes of their own, with no known systemic, or readily identifiable local cause.

They are usually responsible for moderate, to severe, nagging headaches that keeps on recurring.

Due to their habitual recurrence, they are likely to be what people have when they make statements such as this:

"Headache is MY USUAL sickness."

Also, because of how severe and debilitating they can be, they can be easily mistaken for migraines, especially by the uninitiated.

Headache syndromes that fall into this category include;

1. Migraine Headaches

2. Cluster Headaches

3.   Tension   Headaches

4

MIGRAINE

Migraine is more than just headaches: it is a complex neurological disorder usually characterized by warning signs—called prodrome or aura, which culminate in a moderate to severe headache with characteristic features.

Migraines are commoner in adolescents and young adults—especially those that are females. As a rule of the thumb, any headache that started after age 40 to 50 is UNLIKELY a migraine headache.

It is important to note that what makes a headache a Migraine headache, or not, is not the severity of the headache, but its UNIQUE characteristics.

5

RECOGNIZING A MIGRAINE HEADACHE:

Migraines are usually characterized by the following **features**:

✓ A moderate to severe headache.

✓ Headache is usually one-sided. That is, it usually involves just one side of the head, and face [can involve the two sides in some cases, though]. Areas usually involved are the forehead, the sides of the head, and sometimes the neck.

✓ Headache is usually pulsatile, or throbbing.

✓ It is worsened by physical activity: a sufferer would prefer to lie still as even the slightest physical exertion may worsen it.

✓ It may be accompanied by redness of the eyes, and aversion to bright light, and or sound.

✓ It may be accompanied by nausea, and or vomiting.

✓ An episode typically lasts about 4 to 72 hours.

✓ It may come with a premonition, in the form of mood changes, loss of appetite, or nausea.

✓ It is usually preceded by an aura, in some patients. The aura may come as billows of colored lights, or black spots, in the field of vision.

If your Headache does not have at least 70% of these features, if is UNLIKELY   a   Migraine.

6

CLUSTER HEADACHES

These are about the most painful of the primary headaches, more painful than the migraines! As a matter of fact, some schools of thought have it that Clusters may be one of the most painful — if not THE most painful—medical conditions!

The distinguishing hallmark of Clusters is the presence of autonomic symptoms. Thus it is otherwise called Trigeminal AUTONOMIC Cephalalgia.

Cluster headaches are commoner in young males, between the ages 20 to 40.

7

RECOGNIZING A CLUSTER HEADACHE:

Clusters, like Migraine, are usually one-sided.

- Unlike Migraines, however;

✓ The pain is usually around the eyes, and the temple. The patient may feel as if the eyes are being torn out.

✓ They don't switch sides. This means that it usually keeps recurring on the same side of the face. Unlike migraines that can happen on one side of the face in a particular attack, and then on the other side in the next attack.

✓ Clusters last for a shorter duration of time— about 30 minutes to 3 hours. However, they may occur multiple number of times in a day.

✓ The sufferer feels restless, may be pacing about, and may even feel like hitting the head on a wall, unlike in migraines where they prefer to lay still.

- Clusters following a diurnal variation, and usually occur at night.

- They are usually accompanied by autonomic symptoms on the same side of the face as the headache.

This may include;

✓ Redness of the eye

✓ Tearing up

✓ Stuffiness of a nostril, or a runny nose.

✓ Sweating on one side of the face

✓ Drooping eye lid, and narrowed pupil

- Clusters happen multiple number of times in a given period, say over 1 month to 3 months; then gives the patient a long duration of period, say 6 months to a year, without attacks. The attacks come in clusters,   hence   the   name.

8

TENSION HEADACHE

These are the commonest forms of primary headaches, and may even be the commonest cause of headache considering all etiologies, including the secondary types.

Tension headache is the headache you get when you've had a busy day, all stressed up, and perhaps didn't sleep well.

9

RECOGNIZING A TENSION HEADACHE:

✓ It is bilateral. This means that it usually involves the two sides of the head.

✓ It spreads across the forehead, the back of the head, and may also involve the neck, and shoulders.

✓ The sufferer feels a tightness in the head— like there's a tight band tied across their head, or like there's vice-like grip on the head.

✓ It does not possess any of the peculiar features described for the other two types of primary headaches.

10

ON MIGRAINES: RISK FACTORS

*F*actors *that predisposes one to developing a migraine, or that may trigger an attack, include:*

- Drinking of alcohol, especially red wine.

- Flashes of light

- Rapid weather changes

- Skipping of meals

- Stress

- Menses

- Oral contraceptive pills.

-   Etc

11

VARIANTS OF MIGRAINE HEADACHE

These are forms of migraine which— in addition to the symptoms mentioned in the main post— may also come with atypical features.

They include:

1. Hemiplegic Migraine

In which one may be paralyzed on one side of the body during the attack.

2. Ophthalmoplegic Migraine

In which one may have paralysis of the eye muscles.

3. Basilar Migraine

In which one may find it difficult to talk, may have ringing in the ears, and problem maintaining balance.

12

PREVENTION AND TREATMENT

Avoiding the aforementioned triggers as much as possible may help in preventing Migraine attacks.

For people with frequently recurring episodes, oral medications like Beta Blockers, Calcium Channel Blockers, and TCAs, may be used as prophylaxis [Sorry, I'm not writing the exact drug names in order to discourage self-medication].

Mild to moderate attacks can be treated with common analgesics, including NSAIDS, while severe attacks may be treated with Ergot alkaloids, and Triptans.

13

ON CLUSTER: VARIANTS

Variants Of Clusters Headache

- Chronic Paroxysmal Hemicrania

-                          Hemicrania   Continua

14

PREVENTION AND TREATMENT

Calcium Channel Blockers, Mood Stabilizers, and Anticonvulsants may be used for prevention.

NSAIDs may be used to relieve pain.

Acute attacks however needs be aborted with Triptans,or Ergot alkaloids, or Oxygen therapy, or a combination of these.

15

ON TENSION: TYPES

- Episodic Tension Headache

Occurs usually after a stressful day, is mild, and may resolve without treatment.

- Chronic Tension Headache

Occurs almost daily, and is usually more severe.

16

TREATMENT AND PREVENTION

Rest. Exercise. Good eating habit. May all help prevent this type of headache.

Treatment is usually with the over-the-counter analgesics.

www.ingramcontent.com/pod-product-compliance
Lightning Source LLC
Chambersburg PA
CBHW070232260726
48658CB00006BA/2299